The Ultimate Guide to Managing Spinal Stenosis: An Innovative Approach to Effective Management

Louisa Smith

Table of contents

Introduction

Chapter 1 6
Understanding Spinal Stenosis: Symptoms,
Causes, and Types

Chapter 2 8
Diagnosing Spinal Stenosis: Tests and Imaging
Studies

Chapter 3 16
Surgical Options for Spinal Stenosis:
Decompression and Fusion Surgery

Chapter 4 21
Post-operative Care for Spinal Stenosis:
Recovery, Rehabilitation, and Precautions

Chapter 5 25
Alternative Therapies for Spinal Stenosis:
Acupuncture, Chiropractic, and Massage

Chapter 6 29

Lifestyle Changes for Managing Spinal Stenosis: Exercise, Diet, and Stress Management

Chapter 7 34
Coping with Chronic Pain: Emotional and Psychological Aspects of Spinal Stenosis

Chapter 8 38
Managing Spinal Stenosis in Daily Life: Tips for Maintaining Physical Function and Reducing Pain

Chapter 9 41
The Future of Spinal Stenosis Management: Emerging Technologies and Treatments.

Introduction

Spinal stenosis is a condition in which the spinal canal narrows, causing pressure on the spinal cord and nerves. This can lead to symptoms such as pain, numbness, tingling, and muscle weakness in the legs, arms, or lower back. Spinal stenosis can be caused by a variety of factors, including aging, arthritis, spinal injuries, and congenital spinal abnormalities. Treatment options for spinal stenosis may include physical therapy, pain management, and in severe cases, surgery.

Spinal stenosis is a common condition that affects the spinal canal, which is the hollow space in the center of the spine that contains the spinal cord and nerves. The spinal canal is surrounded by bones (vertebrae) and intervertebral discs that protect and cushion the spinal cord.

However, as people age, the bones and discs can begin to degenerate, leading to the formation of bone spurs, herniated discs, or other growths that can narrow the spinal canal and put pressure on the spinal cord and nerves. This can cause a variety of symptoms, including:

Pain, numbness, or tingling in the legs, arms, or lower back
Weakness in the legs, arms, or back
Difficulty walking or standing for long periods of time
Decreased bladder or bowel control (in severe cases)
Treatment options for spinal stenosis depend on the severity of the condition and the specific symptoms experienced. In many cases, physical therapy, pain management, and lifestyle modifications can help manage the symptoms. In more severe cases, surgery may be recommended to relieve the pressure on the spinal cord and nerves and improve symptoms.

It's important for people with symptoms of spinal stenosis to seek medical evaluation, as early diagnosis and treatment can help slow the progression of the condition and improve quality of life.

Chapter 1

Understanding Spinal Stenosis: Symptoms, Causes, and Types

It can cause a range of symptoms, including:

Pain, numbness, or weakness in the legs, arms, or back
Difficulties with balance or coordination
Muscle cramping or fatigue during physical activity
There are several causes of spinal stenosis, including:

Aging and wear and tear on the spine
Inherited conditions that affect the structure of the spine
Herniated discs, bone spurs, or tumors that narrow the spinal canal
Injuries to the spine, such as fractures

There are two main types of spinal stenosis: cervical stenosis, which affects the neck, and lumbar stenosis, which affects the lower back. Treatment options for spinal stenosis vary depending on the severity of the condition, but may include physical therapy, pain medication, or in severe cases, surgery.

Chapter 2

Diagnosing Spinal Stenosis: Tests and Imaging Studies

Diagnosing spinal stenosis typically involves a combination of physical examination, medical history review, and diagnostic tests. Common tests used to diagnose spinal stenosis include:

X-rays: X-rays can show the spinal column and any bony abnormalities, but they cannot show the spinal cord or nerves.

Magnetic Resonance Imaging (MRI): MRI is the most common imaging test used to diagnose spinal stenosis. It provides detailed images of the spinal cord, nerves, and soft tissues, and can show the extent and severity of the stenosis.

Computed Tomography (CT) scan: CT scans can provide detailed images of the bones in the spinal column and can show if there is any compression on the nerves.

Myelogram: A myelogram is a special type of X-ray that uses dye injected into the spinal canal to enhance the images and show the extent of stenosis.

Electromyogram (EMG) and nerve conduction studies: These tests measure the electrical activity of the nerves and muscles and can help determine if there is nerve damage caused by spinal stenosis.

A physical examination may also be conducted to assess symptoms, such as pain, tingling, or weakness, and check for loss of reflexes or muscle weakness. The doctor may also perform tests, such as straight leg raising, to assess nerve function.

It is important to note that the appropriate test or combination of tests will depend on the individual's specific symptoms and medical

history. An accurate diagnosis is crucial for determining the most appropriate course of treatment for spinal stenosis.

In addition to the above tests, other diagnostic procedures that may be used to diagnose spinal stenosis include:

Discography: This is a diagnostic test that involves injecting dye into the intervertebral discs in the spinal column to determine if a particular disc is causing pain.

Flexion-Extension X-rays: This test involves taking X-rays of the spinal column while the patient is bending forward and backward to assess the stability of the spine and determine if there is any spinal cord compression.

Bone scan: A bone scan is a type of imaging test that uses a small amount of radioactive material to help identify areas of abnormal bone activity. This test can be used to help diagnose spinal

stenosis and determine if there is any damage
to the bones in the spinal column.

Overall, the diagnostic tests used to diagnose
spinal stenosis are non-invasive and generally
safe. They are designed to provide a clear
picture of the spinal column and surrounding
structures and help the doctor determine the
best course of treatment for each patient.

In some cases, spinal stenosis can be diagnosed
with a physical examination alone, but more
often, a combination of tests is used to confirm
the diagnosis and determine the extent of the
stenosis. Once a diagnosis is made, the doctor
can develop a treatment plan tailored to the
individual's specific needs and condition.

Non-surgical Treatments for Spinal Stenosis:
Pain Management, Physical Therapy, and
Medications

Non-surgical methods for treating spinal
stenosis include:

Physical therapy: exercises to improve posture,
flexibility, and strength can help relieve
symptoms.

Pain medication: over-the-counter pain
relievers or prescription medication can help
manage pain and inflammation.

Injections: corticosteroid injections can be used
to reduce inflammation and relieve pain in the
affected area.

Lifestyle changes: maintaining a healthy
weight, avoiding activities that exacerbate
symptoms, and using proper body mechanics
can help manage symptoms.

Heat/cold therapy: applying heat or cold to the affected area can help reduce pain and improve mobility.

Bracing: wearing a back brace can help alleviate pressure on the spinal cord and nerves.

It's important to consult a doctor or a specialist to determine the best course of treatment for your specific condition.

Pain Management for spinal stenosis:
Spinal stenosis is a condition that causes pain and discomfort due to the narrowing of the spinal canal. Pain management options include physical therapy, medications, nerve blocks, epidural injections, and sometimes surgery. Physical therapy can help strengthen the muscles surrounding the affected area and improve flexibility, thus reducing pain. Medications such as nonsteroidal anti-inflammatory drugs (NSAIDs), muscle relaxants, and opioids can provide relief from

pain, although they should be used under the guidance of a doctor.

Physical Therapy for spinal stenosis:
Physical therapy is an important part of the treatment plan for spinal stenosis. It can help improve flexibility, strength, and balance, as well as reduce pain. Physical therapy exercises may include stretching, strengthening, and low-impact activities such as walking and swimming. Physical therapy can also help reduce the need for pain medications and improve overall quality of life.

Medications for spinal stenosis:
Medications are commonly used to relieve pain and discomfort associated with spinal stenosis. Over-the-counter pain relievers such as ibuprofen and acetaminophen can be helpful for mild to moderate pain. For more severe pain, prescription medications may be necessary, including nonsteroidal anti-inflammatory drugs (NSAIDs), muscle relaxants, and opioids. It's important to note that these medications can have side effects and

should only be used under the guidance of a doctor.

In summary, spinal stenosis can cause pain and discomfort, and a multi-disciplinary approach to treatment that includes pain management, physical therapy, and medication can help improve quality of life. It's important to work closely with a doctor or healthcare provider to determine the best course of treatment for your individual needs.

Chapter 3

Surgical Options for Spinal Stenosis: Decompression and Fusion Surgery

Spinal stenosis is a condition in which the spinal canal narrows and compresses the spinal cord and/or nerve roots. This can cause pain, numbness, and weakness in the lower back, legs, and/or arms. Surgical options for spinal stenosis include decompression surgery and fusion surgery.

Decompression surgery involves removing the structures that are compressing the spinal cord or nerve roots. This can include removing a portion of a vertebral lamina (laminectomy), removing a portion of a herniated disc (discectomy), or removing a portion of a bone spur (foraminotomy). The goal of decompression surgery is to relieve pressure on the spinal cord or nerve roots and improve symptoms.

Fusion surgery involves joining two or more vertebral bodies together to create a single, solid bone. This is done to stabilize the spine and prevent movement between the affected vertebral segments. Fusion surgery may be done in combination with decompression surgery or as a standalone procedure. The most common type of fusion surgery is an anterior lumbar interbody fusion (ALIF), in which the fusion is performed through the front of the lower back.

Both decompression and fusion surgery can be effective treatments for spinal stenosis, but they also carry risks and potential complications, such as bleeding, infection, nerve damage, and hardware failure. The choice of surgical option depends on several factors, including the location and severity of stenosis, the presence of other spinal problems, and the patient's age and overall health.

It is important to consult with a spine specialist to determine the best surgical option for your individual needs and to fully understand the potential benefits and risks of each procedure.

In addition to decompression and fusion surgery, there are also minimally invasive surgical options for spinal stenosis. These procedures use small incisions and specialized instruments to access the spinal column and decompress the compressed nerves. Minimally invasive surgery typically results in less blood loss, less tissue damage, and a quicker recovery time compared to traditional open surgery.

Examples of minimally invasive surgical options for spinal stenosis include:

Microdecompression: This procedure involves using a small microscope to visualize the compressed nerves and remove the compressing structures using small instruments.

Endoscopic decompression: This procedure involves using a small camera and specialized instruments to access the spinal canal through a small incision and remove the compressing structures.

Percutaneous laser discectomy: This procedure involves using a laser to remove a portion of a herniated disc that is compressing the spinal cord or nerve roots.

The choice between open surgery and minimally invasive surgery will depend on the specific condition and anatomy of the patient.

In conclusion, surgical options for spinal stenosis can vary greatly depending on the specific condition and anatomy of the patient. It is important to consult with a spine specialist to determine the best surgical option for your individual needs and to fully understand the potential benefits and risks of each procedure. Regardless of the chosen surgical option, a thorough preoperative evaluation, a carefully planned surgical technique, and a structured

postoperative rehabilitation program are
critical for optimal outcomes.

Chapter 4

Post-operative Care for Spinal Stenosis: Recovery, Rehabilitation, and Precautions

Post-operative care for spinal stenosis is important for proper recovery and rehabilitation. The following steps should be taken:

Pain management: Pain medication and physical therapy can help manage pain and reduce inflammation after surgery.

Physical therapy: Physical therapy helps to regain strength and flexibility in the back, neck, and legs. It may include exercises to improve mobility, relieve pain, and reduce the risk of future injury.

Precautions: Patients should avoid heavy lifting, bending, and twisting for several weeks after surgery. They should also avoid activities that put too much pressure on the spinal cord, such as running or jumping.

Monitoring for complications: Patients should monitor for any signs of infection, such as fever or increased pain, and report any changes to their doctor immediately.

Adhering to follow-up appointments: Regular follow-up appointments with the doctor help to ensure proper healing and monitor for any complications.

It is important for patients to follow their doctor's instructions and to keep all post-operative appointments. With proper care and rehabilitation, most patients are able to resume their normal activities and enjoy a significant improvement in their quality of life after spinal stenosis surgery.

In addition to the steps mentioned above, here are some other aspects of post-operative care for spinal stenosis:

Adequate rest and sleep: Getting enough sleep and rest helps the body recover from surgery and reduces the risk of complications.

Controlled movements: Controlled movements, such as getting in and out of bed or sitting in a chair, can help prevent injury and reduce pain.

Gradual return to activities: Gradual return to physical activity, as directed by a doctor or physical therapist, helps to prevent re-injury and promotes healing.

Medications: Prescription pain medications may be necessary to manage pain and control inflammation. Over-the-counter pain relievers, such as acetaminophen, may also be recommended.

Avoiding smoking: Smoking can slow down the healing process and increase the risk of complications, such as infections and blood clots.

Maintaining a healthy diet: Eating a well-balanced diet, rich in vitamins and minerals, can help support the body's healing process and improve overall health.

Post-operative care for spinal stenosis is crucial for a successful recovery and rehabilitation. Patients should follow their doctor's instructions, engage in physical therapy, and make lifestyle changes to promote healing and reduce the risk of complications. With proper care, patients can expect to experience significant relief from pain and improved mobility after spinal stenosis surgery.

Chapter 5

Alternative Therapies for Spinal Stenosis: Acupuncture, Chiropractic, and Massage

Acupuncture, chiropractic, and massage are alternative therapies that are sometimes used to help manage symptoms of spinal stenosis.

Acupuncture involves the insertion of thin needles into specific points on the body to stimulate the flow of energy, or "qi." It is thought to help relieve pain and promote healing.

Chiropractic care involves manual adjustments to the spine, with the aim of improving spinal function and reducing pain.

Massage therapy uses hands-on techniques to relieve muscle tension, reduce pain and improve circulation.

It is important to note that while these therapies may provide some relief, they are not a substitute for conventional medical care and should not be used as the sole treatment for spinal stenosis. Consult a doctor to determine the best course of treatment for you.

Acupuncture: This therapy is based on traditional Chinese medicine and has been used for thousands of years to treat various conditions. It is thought that by stimulating specific points on the body, acupuncture can help balance the flow of energy and promote healing. In the case of spinal stenosis, acupuncture may be used to relieve pain, improve flexibility, and reduce inflammation. Research on the effectiveness of acupuncture for spinal stenosis is limited, but some studies suggest that it may be helpful for reducing pain and improving quality of life.

Chiropractic: Chiropractic care is based on the belief that the health of the body is closely linked to the health of the spine. Chiropractors use manual adjustments, also called manipulations, to correct any misalignments in the spine. This is thought to relieve pressure on the nerves and improve spinal function. While there is limited evidence on the effectiveness of chiropractic care for spinal stenosis, some people find it helpful for reducing pain and improving mobility.

Massage: Massage therapy involves the use of different techniques, such as kneading, tapping, and stroking, to manipulate the muscles and soft tissues of the body. It is thought that massage can help relieve muscle tension, reduce pain, and improve circulation. While there is limited research on the effectiveness of massage for spinal stenosis, some people find it helpful for reducing pain and improving mobility.

It's important to note that while these alternative therapies may provide some relief, they are not a substitute for conventional medical care and should not be used as the sole treatment for spinal stenosis. It's also important to consult with a doctor to determine the best course of treatment for you and to ensure that your condition is properly managed.

Chapter 6

Lifestyle Changes for Managing Spinal Stenosis: Exercise, Diet, and Stress Management

To manage spinal stenosis, lifestyle changes such as regular exercise, a balanced diet, and stress management can be helpful.

Exercise:
Low-impact exercises such as walking, swimming, or yoga can help improve flexibility, strengthen the back and legs, and reduce symptoms. Avoid exercises that put strain on the lower back, such as heavy lifting or high-impact activities.

Diet:

A balanced diet rich in nutrients and low in processed foods and sugar can help support overall health and reduce inflammation. Maintaining a healthy weight can also relieve pressure on the spine.

A diet for a patient with spinal stenosis should aim to maintain a healthy weight, reduce inflammation, and provide adequate nutrition to support the healing process. Some recommended dietary guidelines include:

Anti-inflammatory foods: Foods rich in antioxidants, such as berries, leafy greens, and fatty fish, can help reduce inflammation and promote healing.

Fiber-rich foods: Foods high in fiber, such as fruits, vegetables, whole grains, and legumes, can promote digestive health and maintain a healthy weight.

Lean protein: Foods high in lean protein, such as chicken, fish, and tofu, can provide the building blocks for tissue repair and maintenance.

Calcium and Vitamin D: Adequate calcium and vitamin D intake is important for maintaining strong bones and may help reduce the risk of spinal fractures. Foods such as dairy products, leafy greens, and fortified foods are good sources of calcium. Vitamin D can be obtained through exposure to sunlight, as well as through foods like fatty fish and fortified dairy products.

Omega-3 fatty acids: Omega-3 fatty acids have anti-inflammatory properties and can help reduce pain and improve joint mobility. Good sources include fatty fish, such as salmon and mackerel, as well as plant-based sources like flaxseeds and chia seeds.

Herbs and spices: Certain herbs and spices, such as turmeric and ginger, have anti-inflammatory properties and can help reduce pain and improve symptoms of spinal stenosis.

Avoid food triggers: Some people with spinal stenosis may experience increased pain after consuming certain foods. Common food triggers include caffeine, alcohol, and high-fat or high-salt foods. It's a good idea to keep a food diary to identify any potential triggers and avoid them.

Hydration: Staying hydrated is important for overall health and can also help reduce inflammation and improve symptoms of spinal stenosis.

It's also important to limit or avoid processed and junk foods, which can be high in unhealthy fats, added sugars, and salt.

It's important to keep in mind that everyone is unique, and what works for one person may not work for another. It's always a good idea to speak with a healthcare professional or a registered dietitian to determine the best dietary approach for you.

It's always a good idea to speak with a healthcare professional or a registered dietitian before making any major changes to your diet. They can provide individualized recommendations based on your specific health needs and conditions.

Stress Management:
Stress can worsen symptoms of spinal stenosis, so it's important to find ways to manage stress effectively. Techniques such as mindfulness, deep breathing, or regular exercise can help reduce stress and improve overall well-being.

Note: It's important to consult a doctor before making any significant lifestyle changes or starting a new exercise program.

Chapter 7

Coping with Chronic Pain: Emotional and Psychological Aspects of Spinal Stenosis

Chronic pain, particularly spinal stenosis, can have significant emotional and psychological impacts on individuals. Here are some aspects of coping with chronic pain:

Emotional Responses: People with chronic pain often experience emotional symptoms such as depression, anxiety, and frustration. These emotional responses can be due to the constant pain and discomfort, as well as the impact on daily activities and relationships.

Cognitive Changes: Chronic pain can lead to changes in cognitive functioning, including decreased concentration and memory, and increased fatigue.

Impact on Relationships: Chronic pain can impact relationships with friends, family, and intimate partners. It may also lead to feelings of isolation and loneliness.

Coping Strategies: There are several strategies to help cope with the emotional and psychological impacts of chronic pain, including exercise, mindfulness and meditation, counseling, and support groups.

It is important for individuals with chronic pain to address these emotional and psychological aspects, in addition to seeking treatment for the physical pain. A multidisciplinary approach, involving medical professionals, psychologists, and support networks, can help individuals with spinal stenosis effectively manage the physical and emotional aspects of their condition.

Additionally, it is important for individuals with chronic pain to educate themselves about their condition and to understand that their emotional responses are normal and common among people in similar situations. Seeking support from loved ones and participating in support groups can also provide comfort and validation, as well as the opportunity to connect with others who understand the challenges of chronic pain.

It is also essential to have realistic expectations and to avoid pushing oneself too hard. Setting achievable goals and prioritizing self-care can help individuals maintain their emotional and physical well-being.

It is important to note that some people with chronic pain may also benefit from medications to manage their emotional symptoms, such as depression and anxiety. Antidepressants and anti-anxiety medications can help alleviate emotional distress and improve quality of life.

Coping with chronic pain, particularly spinal stenosis, requires a comprehensive approach that addresses the emotional and psychological impacts. With the right support and resources, individuals can learn to manage their symptoms and maintain a positive outlook despite the challenges posed by chronic pain.

Chapter 8

Managing Spinal Stenosis in Daily Life: Tips for Maintaining Physical Function and Reducing Pain

Spinal stenosis is a condition that affects the spine and can cause discomfort, pain and reduced mobility. To manage spinal stenosis in daily life, one can follow the following tips:

Exercise regularly: Light exercises like walking, swimming, or yoga can help keep the spine flexible and improve circulation. Avoid high-impact exercises that put too much stress on the spine.

Maintain a healthy weight: Excess weight puts extra strain on the spine, so maintaining a healthy weight is important to reduce pain and prevent further damage.

Good posture: Maintaining good posture when standing, sitting, or walking helps distribute weight evenly and reduce strain on the spine.

Avoid prolonged periods of sitting or standing: Alternating between sitting and standing every 30 minutes can reduce the pressure on the spine and improve circulation.

Use heat or ice: Applying heat or ice to the affected area can help relieve pain and reduce inflammation.

Medications: Over-the-counter pain medications like ibuprofen and acetaminophen can help relieve symptoms.

Physical therapy: A physical therapist can develop a personalized exercise program to help improve mobility and reduce pain.

Surgery: In severe cases, surgery may be necessary to relieve pressure on the spinal cord.

It is important to remember that everyone's experience with spinal stenosis is different, and what works for one person may not work for another. If symptoms persist or worsen, it's important to seek medical advice.

Chapter 9

The Future of Spinal Stenosis Management: Emerging Technologies and Treatments.

Spinal stenosis is a common condition characterized by the narrowing of the spinal canal, which can lead to pain and nerve damage. The management of spinal stenosis has advanced significantly in recent years, with new technologies and treatments emerging that aim to improve patient outcomes and quality of life.

One of the most promising technologies in spinal stenosis management is minimally invasive surgery. These procedures use smaller incisions, which results in less scarring, faster recovery times, and less risk of complications compared to traditional open surgery.

Another emerging technology is the use of regenerative medicine, including stem cell therapy and platelet-rich plasma (PRP) injections. These treatments aim to repair damaged tissue and reduce inflammation, leading to improved pain relief and reduced need for medication.

Image-guided technology, such as computer-assisted navigation and intraoperative imaging, is also becoming more widely used in spinal stenosis management. This technology helps surgeons to accurately locate and treat the affected areas with greater precision, resulting in better patient outcomes.

Physical therapy, exercise, and weight management can also play a crucial role in managing spinal stenosis. These non-invasive approaches can help to improve flexibility, strength, and stability, reducing the risk of further injury and the need for surgery.

The future of spinal stenosis management is looking promising, with a range of emerging

technologies and treatments that offer
improved patient outcomes and reduced risk of
complications. However, it is important to seek
the advice of a qualified healthcare professional
to determine the best course of treatment for
each individual case.

In addition to the technologies and treatments
mentioned above, there are several other
emerging developments in the field of spinal
stenosis management.

One of these is the use of radiofrequency
ablation, which uses heat to target and destroy
nerve tissue that is causing pain. This
minimally invasive procedure has been shown
to be effective in reducing pain and improving
quality of life for many patients with spinal
stenosis.

Another promising development is the use of
spinal cord stimulation, which involves the
placement of electrodes near the spinal cord to
deliver electrical impulses and reduce pain.
This technology is being used increasingly in
the management of chronic pain, including

spinal stenosis, and has been shown to be highly effective in many cases.

Furthermore, new surgical techniques, such as endoscopic spinal surgery, are being developed that aim to provide a more minimally invasive alternative to traditional open surgery.